Zannis

4th edition

obstetrics and gynecology